Geriatric Symptom Assessment and Management

Cardiopulmonary

Kathleen Ryan Fletcher, RN, CS, MSN, GNP

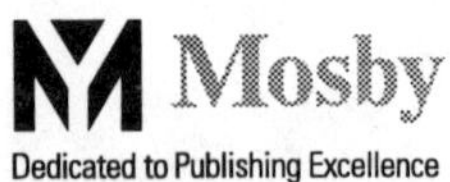

Dedicated to Publishing Excellence

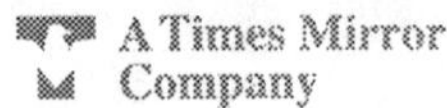

Publisher: Nancy L. Coon
Acquisitions Editor: Jacqueline Katz
Editor: Loren Wilson
Developmental Editor: Glenn Floyd
Project Supervisor: Gayle Morris
Cover Design: Laura Eslinger, The Painted Page
Manufacturing Supervisor: Pam Morris

Printed in the United States of America
Printing/binding by Plus Communications

Mosby, Inc.
11830 Westline Industrial Drive
St. Louis, Missouri 63146

International Standard Book Number 0-8151-2697-2

97 98 99 00 01 / 9 8 7 6 5 4 3 2 1

REVIEWERS

Doris Ballard-Ferguson, PhD, APN-GNP
Associate Professor
Graduate Specialty Coordinator
Gerontological Nurse Practitioner Specialty
College of Nursing
University of Arkansas for Medical Sciences
Little Rock, Arkansas

Priscilla Ebersole, PhD, RN, FAAN
Editor, *Geriatric Nursing*

Annette Lueckenotte, MS, RN, CS
Gerontological Nurse Practitioner
Alexian Brothers Senior Health Center
St. Louis, Missouri

Ann Schmidt Luggen, PhD, RN, CNAA
Associate Professor, Nursing
Northern Kentucky University
Highland Heights, Kentucky
Vice President
National Gerontological Nursing Association

PREFACE

Geriatric Symptom Assessment and Management

The Geriatric Symptom Assessment and Management video/workbook series teaches the nurse how to incorporate the knowledge of the pathophysiology of a symptom together with the assessment and management of that symptom. The series consists of four videotapes and their accompanying workbooks. Module One presents a framework for symptom assessment and clinical decision making in geriatric care. The remaining modules/workbooks illustrate how this framework is applied with common geriatric symptoms. Unlike the traditional assessment approach that teaches nurses how to do a complete physical exam, this series is designed to help nurses conduct a realistic episodic assessment based on a presenting symptom.

In addition, one contact hour is available for each video/booklet title reviewed. The instructions for completing the post-test and receiving continuing education credit are included in the Continuing Education section of each booklet.

ABOUT THE AUTHOR

Kathleen Ryan Fletcher, RN, CS, MSN, GNP, is a gerontological nurse practitioner working in Patient Care Services at the University of Virginia Health Systems in Charlottesville, Virginia. In her role, she is involved in the development, implementation, and evaluation of interdisciplinary geriatric services throughout a continuum of care.

Kathy received her bachelor's degree in nursing from Pennsylvania State University in 1971. She received a master's degree as a gerontological nurse practitioner from the University of Lowell in Lowell, Massachusetts in 1982. Her varied experiences include staff nursing at Temple Hospital in Philadelphia, Pennsylvania, public health nursing at the Veterans Medical Center in Prescott, Arizona, and Associate Chief Nurse for Extended Care ar the Veterans Medical Center in Wilkes Barre, Pennsylvania. While on faculty at the University of Virginia School of Nursing, Kathy set up and managed a nurse-run clinic in low-income housing for the elderly. She remains committed to maintaining a "hands-on" nursing practice role.

Kathy has taught continuing education programs in gerontological nursing throughout the United States and Canada. She is known for her realistic teaching style and case-based approach. She has published extensively and exclusively in gerontological nursing. She is currently President of the National Conference of Gerontological Nurse Practitioners and is Chair of the Board on Credentialing, Gerontological Nursing for the American Nurses Association.

CONTENTS

Geriatric Symptom Assessment and Management

Workbook

OBJECTIVES

After watching the videotape and completing the workbook, viewers will be able to:

- Differentiate between normal aging and signs and symptoms that are indicative of a disease process.
- Understand the pathophysiology and etiology of common symptoms/signs in the older adult.
- Prioritize signs to look for based on symptoms and behavioral cues presented by the older individual.
- Determine whether the clinical presentation of a symptom or sign is an emergent, urgent, or non-urgent situation.
- Collect data from communication-impaired older adults.
- Discuss common atypical presentations in the older adults and their significance.
- Define symptom management strategies for commonly presented symptoms in the elderly.
- Identify presentation strategies important in minimizing the risk that symptoms/signs of illness will develop.

INTRODUCTION

This workbook identifies relevant aging changes that affect cardiopulmonary assessment (Table 2-1). This is followed by a discussion of cardiopulmonary symptoms and signs common in the elderly. These symptoms/signs include edema, chest pain, and dyspnea. For each of these disorders, the pathophysiology of the symptom will be covered followed by a discussion of the possible etiologies. Using the framework described in Module One, a comprehensive symptom evaluation will be detailed. Pharmacological and non-pharmacological symptom management strategies will be presented. With each identified symptom, education and prevention strategies are illustrated.

Table 2-1 Cardiopulmonary Changes with Aging

Cardiovascular Change	Appearance or Functional Change	Implication
Fibrous and thickened heart valves	Possible reduced stroke volume Change in cardiac output Left ventricular hypertrophy	Decreased responsiveness to stress Increased incidence of murmurs
Increase in subpericardial fat		
Collagen accumulation around heart muscle		
Fibroelastic thickening of the SA node	Slower heart rate	Increased prevalence of arrhythmias
Decreased number of pacemaker cells		
Elongation/tortuosity and calcification of arteries	Increase in systolic blood pressure	Possible formation of aneurysms Decrease in blood flow to body organs
Progressive thickening and loss of resiliency of arterial wall	Increasing rigidity of arterial wall	Altered distribution of blood flow Increased incidence of atherosclerosis

| Lipid content increases in artery wall
Decreased baroreceptor sensitivity | Increased peripheral vascular resistance | Tendency to lose balance |

Pulmonary Changes with Aging	**Appearance or Functional Change**	**Implication**
Decrease in elasticity of lung tissue	Decrease in vital capacity Increased residual volume Decrease in maximum breathing capacity	Reduced overall efficiency of ventilatory exchange
Thoracic wall calcification	Increased AP diameter of chest	Obscuration of heart sounds Displacement of apical impulse
Cilial atrophy Decrease in respiratory muscle strength	Reduced ability to handle secretions and reduced effectiveness against noxious foreign particles; or partial inflation of lungs at rest	Increased susceptibility to infection

EDEMA

Edema is defined as an increase in interstitial fluid as a result of the expansion of extracellular fluid volume. Lymphedema is an increase in hydrostatic pressure caused by an accumulation of lymph. Lipedema is an accumulation of fatty tissue.

Pathophysiology: Edema

In the newborn, 80 percent of the total body weight is water. This decreases to about 60 percent in the adult and may decrease to 45 percent in the older adult (Merck, 1995). More important than volume is the actual distribution of this water. Typically, approximately two-thirds is intracellular fluid (ICF) and one-third is extracellular fluid (ECF) (Figure 2-1).

Figure 2-1 Body Water Composition of the Older Adult

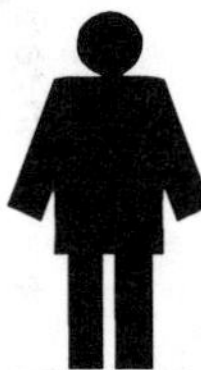

- Total BW = 40 liters

- ICF = 25 liters

- ECF = 15 liters

In the elderly, the loss of water primarily occurs inside the cells. As this happens, the areas outside the cells will therefore attain a greater proportion of the total fluid volume.

Starling's concept of osmotic pressure demonstrates that fluid flows from vessels into the interstitial tissue in response to both intravascular pressure and the colloid osmotic pressure of the interstitial fluid (Figure 2-2).

Figure 2-2 Osmotic Pressure Gradient

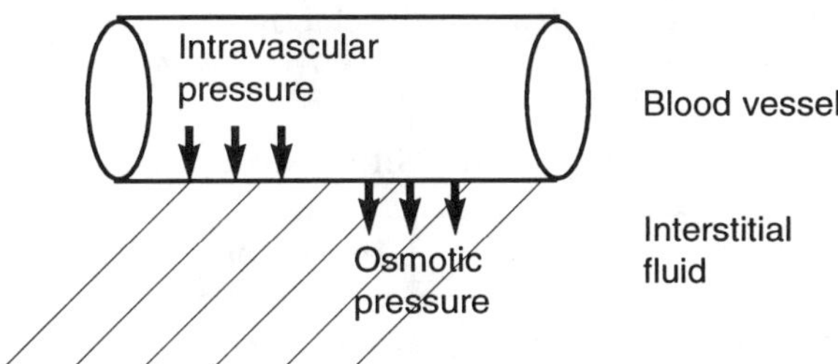

In the opposite direction, fluid enters the blood because of interstitial tissue tension and the oncotic pressure of plasma protein (Figure 2-3).

Figure 2-3 Oncotic Pressure Gradient

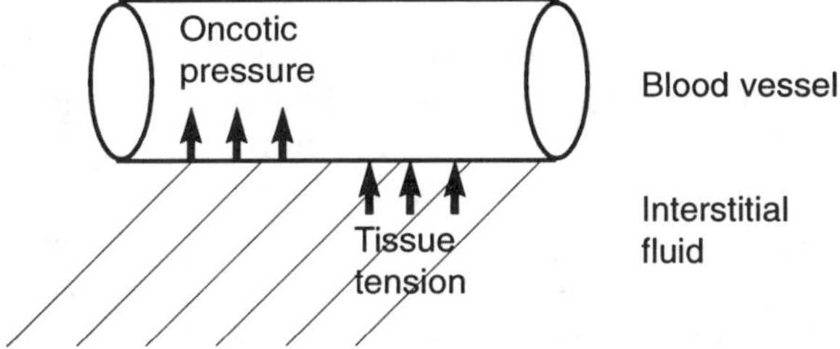

Interstitial fluid is also returned to the blood as lymph. Alteration in any of these components upsets the equilibrium (DeGowin, 1987). Two basic steps occur in edema formation: dietary sodium and water are retained, and capillary hemodynamics are altered.

Etiology: Edema

The causes of edema in the elderly are diverse yet common (Table 2-2).

Table 2-2 Common Causes of Edema in the Elderly

Bilateral	Unilateral
Cardiovascular disease	Venous obstruction
Renal disease	Lymphatic obstruction
Thyroid disease	Inflammation
Liver disease	Infection
Hypoalbuminemia	Tumor
Drug-induced reaction	Trauma
Allergic reaction	

Cardiovascular causes such as chronic venous insufficiency, heart failure, pulmonary hypertension, and valvular dysfunction are frequent in the elderly. Edema due to an increased interstitial volume is often seen with renal failure, liver disease, and hypoalbuminemia. The colloid pressure in plasma is mostly generated by protein, which keeps water in the intravascular space. When the level of protein is reduced, there is a reduction in intravascular oncotic pressure, which subsequently leads to an increase in interstitial volume, and pitting edema occurs (Ciocon, 1993). Medications commonly taken by the elderly may cause edema (Table 2-3).

Table 2-3 Medications That Can Cause Edema

Antihypertensives	Calcium channel blockers, clonodine, hydralazine, methyldopa
Hormones	Cortocosteroids, estrogen, testosterone, progesterone
Nonsteroidal antiinflammatories	Any type

Symptom Evaluation: Edema

The symptom of edema may be vague or nonspecific. The older adult may describe it as a fullness, achy discomfort, or weight gain—or they may say their shoes feel too tight. As with any symptom, it is important for the health care provider to focus on the seven steps of symptom assessment covered in Module One (Table 2-4).

Table 2-4 Seven Dimensions of Symptom Assessment

Location
Severity
Quality
Chronological evolution
Aggravating and alleviating factors
Associated symptoms
Impact on daily life

With edema, the most important questions are location and distribution (unilateral or bilateral), duration and progression (acute or chronic), and accompanying signs and symptoms.

Physical Examination: Edema

Weight:

Note: It is important to weigh the individual at the same time, on the same scale, and with approximately the same weight of clothing.

Skin Changes:

Examine the skin for lesions, discoloration, texture, trophic changes, and induration.

Circulation (arterial and venous):

Look for dependent redness. Elevate the leg until the foot becomes pale. With arterial insufficiency, it becomes a bluish color when elevated; when dependent, it will turn a deep red-blue color. At the same time, note the venous filling time that normally occurs within 10-12 seconds of becoming dependent.

Check pulse points in the extremities, including the femoral, dorsalis pedis, and posterior tibial. Doppler readings may become necessary if there is difficulty in palpating.

Check capillary refill by pressing the distal end of the nail plate and releasing it. Normally it will take less than 5 seconds for a pink flush to return.

Check for tenderness of the extremity:

Note: diffuse or local tenderness.

Check for pitting or nonpitting edema:

Look in the most dependent body area. For example, the patient who has been immobile may have edema at the sacrum.

Note: Pitting is caused by retrograde pressure at the

capillary level. In nonpitting cases, fluid is clotted with fibrinogen and may be called hard or brawny. High-viscosity fluid such as lymphedema is usually nonpitting (Merli, 1995).

Measure circumference:

Note: avoid the use of edema scales.

Measure the exact circumference at a designated point such as the calf or patella. For sequential readings, mark the area with a skin-marking pencil. A difference greater than 1 cm between extremities is considered significant.

Examine the appropriate systems:

This may include cardiac, renal, and endocrine systems, as the history dictates. Diagnostic tests focus on the probable etiology of edema.

Treatment/Management: Edema

Pharmacological management is aimed at the specific disease or process and may be prescribed by the appropriate health care professional (Table 2-5).

Table 2-5 Pharmacological Treatment for Edema

Heart failure: diuretics
Hypoalbuminemia: colloids or high-protein diet
Proteinuria: ace inhibitors
Acute deep venous thrombosis: thrombolytics

Nonpharmacological management is also targeted at the specific process and may include:

- fluid and sodium restriction
  (Note: Water intake is sometimes restricted along with sodium so that a dilutional hyponatremia does not occur.)

- pressure gradient stockings
  (Note: These work for a limited time, and compliance may be a problem)

- compression leg pump
  (Note: This is not recommended in the presence of pain, numbness, severe arteriosclerosis, or massive edema.)

- leg elevation
  (Note: This decreases peripheral vascular pressure.)

- weight reduction, if indicated

Education/Prevention: Edema

Regular exercise, maintaining a healthy weight, and moderate intake of sodium are important in preventing dependent edema. Leg raising exercises done regularly—especially when on long trips—will increase the muscle pump action. Special care of the skin includes wearing proper-sized shoes and providing adequate lubrication. The older adult should be taught to prevent trauma, to prevent the legs from sunburn, and to never apply a heating pad to painful, swollen legs.

CHEST PAIN

Chest pain is one of the most common symptoms among older adults presenting to the emergency room. The complaint of chest pain or even mild discomfort in the elderly may be indicative of a severe life threat. A study published in the *Journal of the American Geriatrics Society* (Bayer, 1986) reflected that in the young old (65-85), the most common symptoms of myocardial infarctions were chest pain and diaphoresis, but in those over age 85, more common symptoms included acute confusion and shortness of breath.

Pathophysiology: Chest Pain

There are many different etiologies of chest pain syndromes. This may be attributed to neurons that cross or overlap. Sensory neurons from most intra-thoracic organs cross the cardiac or pulmonary nerves and sympathetic ganglia on their way to the dorsal thoracic nerve roots. Because of this, it becomes difficult to determine the exact location of the origin of the pain.

Descriptions of chest pain may give clues to the origin. Visceral pain, often referred to as organ pain, is usually described as vague and is characterized by having a dull or aching quality. Cutaneous or surface pain tends to be described as being sharp or tingling in nature.

Etiology: Chest Pain

There are three primary sources of chest pain:
- intrathoracic: heart, lungs, trachea
- extrathoracic: neck, trachea, visceral organs
- psychogenic: anxiety, panic

Possible causes of chest pain are noted in the following figure. (Figure 2-4: Bittner, 1995)

Figure 2-4 Possible Causes of Chest Pain of Unknown Origin

Possible causes of chest pain of unknown origin

The differential diagnosis includes cardiovascular, pulmonary, gastrointestinal, musculoskeletal, neurologic, and psychological sources of pain. The more common conditions are listed below.

Cardiovascular

- Coronary artery disease
- Angina
- Coronary atherosclerosis
- Microvascular
- Prinzmetal's
- Myocardial infarction
- Aortic stenosis
- Hypertensive heart disease
- Hypertrophic cardiomyopathy
- Pericarditis
- Pulmonary hypertension
- Mitral valve prolapse
- Cocaine use

Musculoskeletal

- Cervical disc disease
- Arthritis of the shoulder girdle
- Costochondritis
- Tietze's syndrome
- Intercostal muscle cramps

Psychological

- Panic attacks

Neurologic

- Herpes zoster

Pulmonary

- Pulmonary embolism
- Pneumonia
- Bronchitis
- Pleuritis
- Pneumothorax
- Tumor
- Mediastinal disease

Gastrointestinal

- Esophageal reflux
- Esophagitis
- Esophageal spasm
- Mallory-Weiss tear
- Peptic ulcer disease
- Gallbladder disease
- Pancreatitis

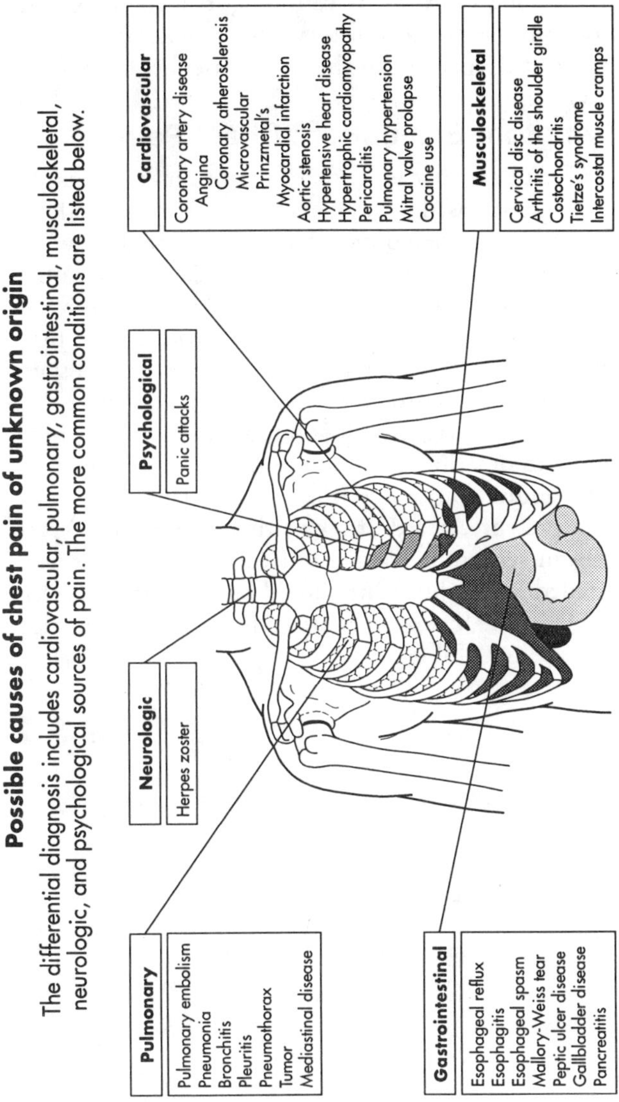

Even the most experienced clinicians have difficulty distinguishing ischemic pain from nonischemic etiologies. In one study where cardiologists made judgments based on the medical history, the cardiologist was incorrect 25 percent of the time (Aisenberg, 1994).

Symptom Evaluation: Chest Pain

Chest pain that is acute, of recent onset, or that has recently increased in frequency or severity, should always be considered unstable and evaluated immediately in the hospital. Older adults with a history of coronary artery disease, displaying changes in the electrocardiogram, experiencing anginal pain at rest, displaying unstable vital signs, or who have mental status changes, should also be evaluated immediately.

When interviewing, it is important to get the individual to describe the discomfort. The majority of older adults do not describe it as pain but rather heaviness, pressure, heartburn, or a tired feeling. The seven steps in symptom evaluation (see Table 2-4) that were detailed in Module One should be used. Specific elements in the history that are to be more detailed are listed below (Table 2-6).

Table 2-6 Chest Pain: Assessment by History

Onset:	trauma relationship, predictable
Aggravating factors:	emotional upset, swallowing, cold weather, sexual intercourse, deep breathing, coughing, neck position change, or movement of the arm or chest
Relieving factors:	food, antacid, nitroglycerine, rest, change of position, massage
Past treatment/evaluation:	electrocardiogram, upper GI, chest x-ray
Associated symptoms:	anxiety, depression, faintness, palpitation, numbness or tingling in hands or around mouth, fever, chills, sweating, syncope, cough, sputum production, hemoptysis, dyspnea, tenderness, swallowing difficulty, nausea, vomiting, leg swelling or pain, weight change
Medical history:	lung disease, chest surgery, chest injury, cardiovascular disease, hypertension, diabetes, elevated cholesterol or triglyceride, angina, phlebitis, emotional problems
Medications:	hormones, diuretics, digitalis, bronchodilators, nitroglycerine, tranquilizers, sedatives, antacids
Family history:	cardiovascular disease, diabetes, hypertension, elevated blood lipids
Environmental history:	smoking, mining, exposure to asbestos

Physical Examination: Chest Pain

General appearance:

Note: Focus on the level of distress.

Vital signs:

Check regularity and quality of pulse. Blood pressure is checked in both arms positionally. Check temperature.

Skin:

Assess moisture, color, capillary refill. Check the lower extremities for temperature changes, tenderness, and edema.

Cardiac:

Look for neck vein distension. Inspect over the valvular areas (Figure 2-5) for lifts or thrusting of the chest wall.

Figure 2-5 Valvular Areas

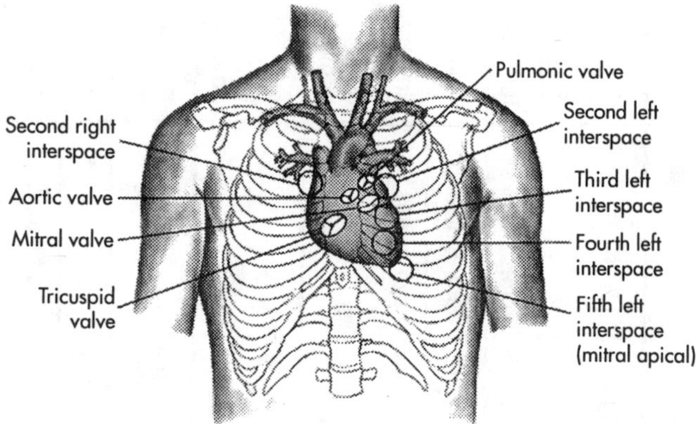

Palpate over the valvular areas (aortic, pulmonic, tricuspid, and mitral) for thrills. Check for displacement of the point of maximal impulse (PMI), which normally is at the fourth or fifth left intercostal space at the midclavicular line.

Auscultate each valvular area with the diaphragm (for high-frequency tones) and the bell (for low-frequency tones). Listen for S1, S2, the systolic interval (between S1 and S2), and the diastolic interval (between S2 and S1). Listen for extra heart sounds and murmurs and pericardial rubs.

Listen to the carotids for bruit.

Pulmonary:

Look at the breathing pattern. Palpate the chest wall for tenderness. Auscultate for adventitious sounds.

Crackles (fluid sounds) are more commonly heard at the bases. Wheezes (constricted airway sounds) may be auscultated anywere. Pleural rub may be heard at the lateral border.

Abdomen:

Check for abdominal distension. Listen for bruit at the abdominal aorta. Auscultate bowel sounds. J3 Palpate for enlarged organs.

Other systems may be examined, as dictated by the history, and might include neuromuscular or skeletal.

Treatment/Management: Chest Pain

Pharmacological management of chest pain is always aimed at the specific disease process and is prescribed by an appropriate health care professional (Table 2-7).

Table 2-7 Pharmacological Managment of Chest Pain

Etiology	Possible Treatment
Ischemia	Calcium channel blockers Nitrates Beta blockers
Costovertebral	Tylenol®
Myocardial infarction	Aspirin Heparin Thrombolytics
Pulmonary embolism	Anticoagulants
Peptic ulcer disease	Antacids Antisecretory Antibiotics
Herpes zoster	Antiviral
Esophageal	H_2 receptor antagonist
Psychogenic	Anxiolytics

Nonpharmacological management also targets the specific etiology for the pain and may include:

- Avoiding stress, heavy meals, and strenuous exercise (for ischemic).

- Weight reduction (for ischemic or nonischemic etiologies), if appropriate.

- Avoiding smoking, alcohol, or caffeine.

- Reducing fat intake and avoiding peppermint (for gastroesophagel reflux etiologies).

- Avoiding late night feeding and keeping the head elevated for 45 minutes after meals.

Education/Prevention: Chest Pain

Maintaining a healthy lifestyle and proper nutrition, exercise, and stress reduction are important in the prevention of cardiovascular disease. Heart-healthy guidelines (Table 2-8) should be followed. Older adults and families are instructed to call an emergency response system for new or changed chest pain.

Table 2-8 Heart-Healthy Guidelines

Get regular exercise.
Maintain proper diet and appropriate body weight.
Control stress.
Stop smoking.
Control cholesterol levels, hypertension, and diabetes.

DYSPNEA

There is no specific or widely accepted definition of dyspnea. The strict interpretation of dyspnea is disordered breathing (Silvestri, 1993), but this does not describe the individual experience. Here it is referred to as the conscious awareness of increased respiratory effort. A healthy person might experience it with extreme exertion, and the chronic obstructive pulmonary patient may experience it with minimal expenditure of effort. It is a complex symptom that arises from a series of steps. There are also different varieties of dyspnea, including orthopnea—which is dyspnea in the recumbent position—and paroxysmal nocturnal dyspnea—which is dyspnea in the recumbent position that is periodic at night.

Pathophysiology: Dyspnea

There are a variety of sensory systems involved in the regulation of breathing. These include chemoreceptors in the blood and the brain and mechanoreceptors in the airway, lungs, and muscles (Figure 2-6: Raffin, 1984).

Figure 2-6 Factors Influencing the Control of Ventilation

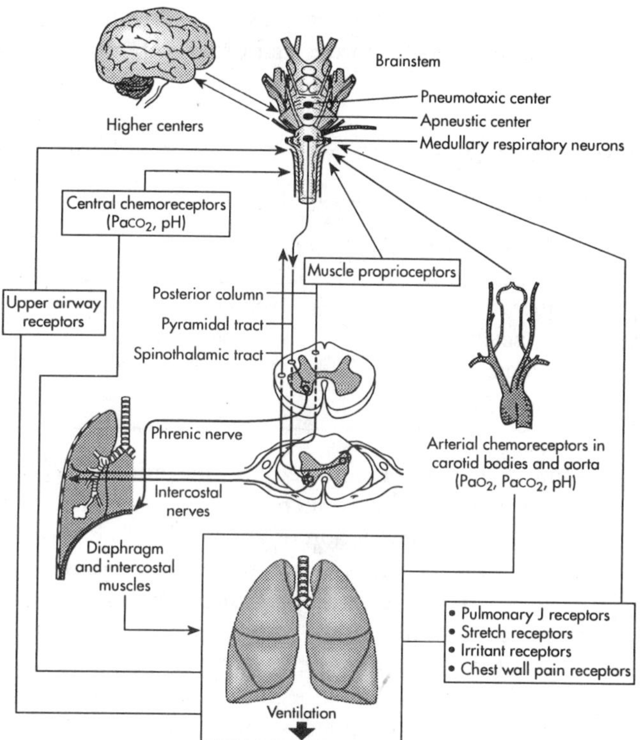

Several pathological mechanisms underlie dyspnea. There could be decreased airflow due to obstruction in the airways, airway narrowing, or airway collapse. There may be a failure of the lungs to meet tissue demands as seen with CO_2 acidosis and certain drugs. The respiratory center in the brain stem can affect ventilatory effort.

Etiology: Dyspnea

Dyspnea can arise from a number of causes (Table 2-9).

Table 2-9 Dyspnea: Possible Causes

Respiratory	Mechanical
Cardiovascular	Psychological
Hematological	Deconditioning
Metabolic	

Pulmonary causes include embolism, pulmonary edema, obstruction due to increased airway resistance (i.e., asthma), and restriction of airflow due to decreased pulmonary compliance. Cardiac causes include mitral valve lesions, thrombus, and pericardial effusion. At times, the cardiac and pulmonary etiologies coexist, of which heart failure is a prime example (Figure 2-7: Raffin, 1984). When the heart begins to fail as a pump, it attempts to maintain cardiac output through increased left ventricular diastolic pressure and volume. This compensation is referred to as the Frank Starling mechanism. Then, as the left atrial, pulmonary venous, and pulmonary capillary pressures are increased, fluid seeps out of the blood vessel and crosses from the pulmonary circulation into the lung tissue. The blood vessel enlargement, coupled with the diminished compliance of congested tissue, adds to the work of breathing and contributes to the sensation of dyspnea.

Figure 2-7 Dyspnea in Cardiac Failure

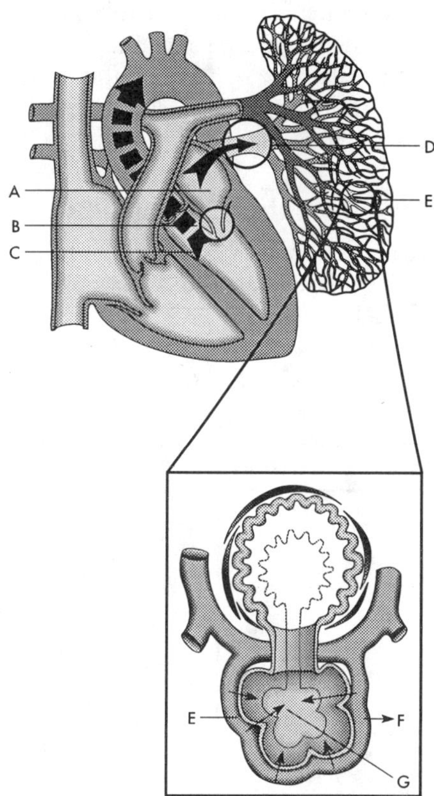

Left atrial (A) pressure elevation occurs as a result of either obstruction at the mitral valve (B) or inadequate emptying of the left ventricle (C). Pulmonary vascular (D) engorgement ensues, producing elevated pulmonary capillary (E) pressure, which leads to transudation of fluid into the interstitial tissue (F), resulting in a less compliant lung. This loss of compliance increases the respiratory effort (dyspnea), which becomes more pronounced as fluid enters the alveolus (G) to manifest clinically as pulmonary edema, in effect, a type of *restrictive lung disease*.

Dyspnea can also be caused by metabolic (thyroid), hematologic (anemia, carbon minoxide), and mechanical factors (enlarged organs, large abdomen). In addition, it can be caused by hyperventilation (anxiety), or it can be drug-induced (beta blocker, benzodiazepine, phenothiazine, narcotic).

Symptom Evaluation: Dyspnea

When the older adult is experiencing respiratory distress, emergency assessment and management is indicated (Table 2-10).

Table 2-10 Emergency Assessment and Management of Dyspnea

Assessment	Management
Check airway.	Clear any obstruction.
Look for cyanosis, low O_2 level.	Administer oxygen.
Check for hyperventilation.	Have person breathe into a paper bag.
Watch for signs of ventilation failure.	Support ventilation.

Ask the individual to describe the breathing sensation. Get a detailed description of the symptom using the framework as a general guide (Table 2-4). With dyspnea, it is always important to identify when the person became aware of the symptom (acute or chronic onset). The frequency and severity of the symptoms are usually interrelated. Helpful tools include the Visual Analogue Scale (Mahler, 1987) and the Borg Dyspnea Rating Scale (Borg, 1982).

Figure 2-8 Dyspnea Scales

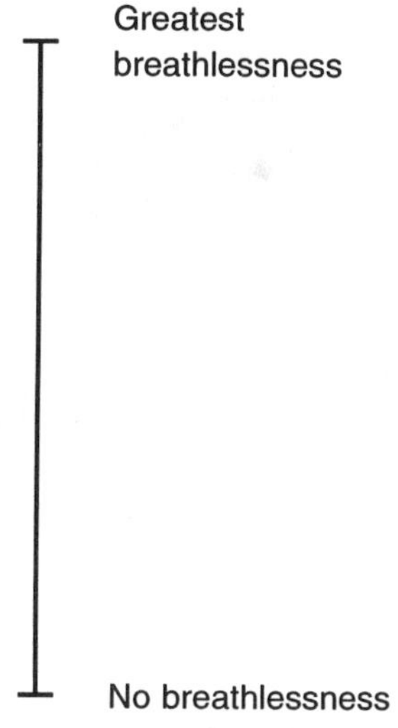

The visual analog scale can be used to measure breathlessness and other symptoms during cardiopulmonary
exercise testing.

(Continued)

Figure 2-8 Dyspnea Scales (cont'd)

0	Nothing at all
0.5	Very, very slight (just noticeable)
1	Very slight
2	Slight (light)
3	Moderate
4	Somewhat severe
5	Severe (heavy)
6	
7	Very severe
8	
9	
10	Very, very severe (almost maximal)
•	Maximal

The 0 to 10 category-ratio scale can be used to measure breathlessness and other symptoms during cardiopulmonary exercise testing.

Look for precipitating factors or events such as weight gain, respiratory infection, new medications, dust, and recent surgery. Ask about exposure to tobacco, inhalants, animals, or birds. Question the individual about associated symptoms such as coughing, fever, chills, edema, sputum production, and pleuretic chest pain. Anxiety and depression are factors often associated with dyspnea (Gift, 1993).

Estimate the disability level by determining how breathlessness affects daily activities. It is important to note that when older adults are frail and deconditioned, they are more likely to experience shortness of breath with activity. It is also important to consider that if older persons typically do not exert themselves, they may not experience the symptom of dyspnea until the underlying disease is extensive.

Physical Examination: Dyspnea

Vital signs:

Look at the rate and depth of respiration and the breathing pattern. Is the individual using accessory muscles or pursed lip breathing?

Check the temperature and weight.

Look for jugular venous distention.

Pulmonary:

Inspect the chest wall for barrel chest. Look for symmetry of movement in the intercostal space.

Palpate the chest for tactile fremitus. Using the flat of the hand in intercostal spaces, have the person say "99." The normal voice produces a palpable vibration.

Percussion:

Compare side to side. A significant finding is dullness where resonance should be present. The normal resting diaphragm is percussed at the 9th rib interspace.

Auscultation (Figure 2-9: Seidel, 1991):

Normal sounds include vesicular (fine, high pitch) in the periphery; bronchial (harsher, coarser) over the trachea, and brochovesicular sounds (a combined sound) over the main stem bronchus. Common adventitous (abnormal) sounds include crackles (fluid sounds) and wheezes (constricted airway sounds).

Figure 2-9 Schema of Breath Sounds in the Well and Ill Patient

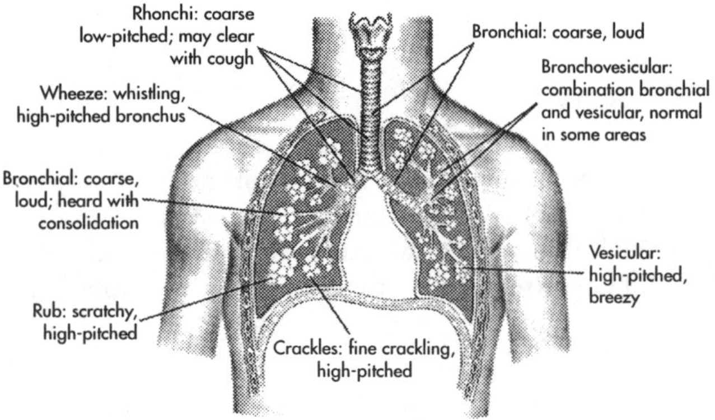

Cardiovascular:

Check for signs of cardiac enlargement, extra heart sounds, or murmurs. Aortic murmurs are best auscultated with the older adult leaning forward and holding the breath in exhalation. Mitral murmurs are best auscultated with the older adult in a left lateral decubitus position while listening over the point of maximal impulse.

Peripheral vascular:

Check for clubbing (Figure 2-10: Seidel, 1991) that is indicative of chronic hypoxia.

Figure 2-10 Clubbing

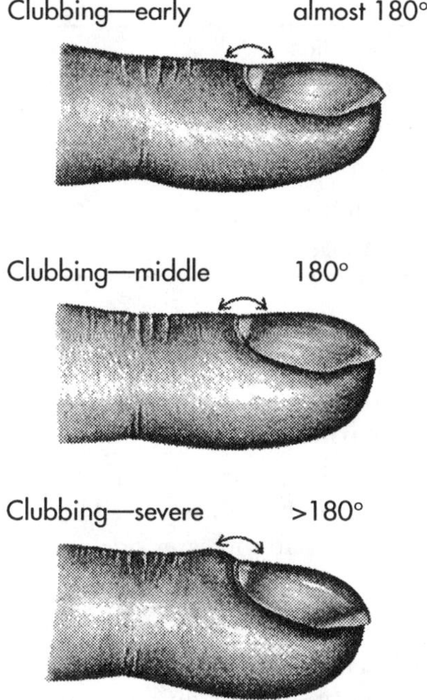

Check capillary refill and determine whether any edema is present.

Abdominal exam:

Check for enlarged organs, masses, or tenderness.

Additional diagnostic testing may include a chest x-ray, electrocardiogram, pulmonary function tests, arterial blood gases, and pulse oximetry (Seamens, 1995).

Treatment/Management: Dyspnea

Pharmacological management is always directed at the cause and prescribed by an appropriate health care professional (Table 2-12).

Table 2-12 Pharmacological Treatment for Dyspnea

Heart failure: diuretics
Bronchoconstriction: bronchodilators
Pneumonia: antibiotics
Hypoxia: oxygen
Anxiety: psychotropics
Anemia: blood replacement

Nonpharmacological measures assist the older adult in managing the symptom of dyspnea.

Pursed lip breathing:

The individual is taught to inspire 1-2 seconds then to exhale 5-10 seconds against pursed lips. This slows the respiratory rate and increases tidal volume.

Diaphragmatic breathing:

The individual is taught first to relax the abdominal wall during inspiration, allowing more unobstructed descent of the diaphragm. Then the individual is taught to tighten the abdomen during expiration, thus enhancing the upward movment of the diaphragm.

General muscle training:

This increases exercise tolerance.

Pacing activities:

Chronic dyspnic individuals are taught to pace themselves and to allow frequent rest periods, and they are encouraged to transfer some activities to others.

Proper nutrition:

Note: Higher carbohydrate diets result in increased CO_2 production and can worsen ventilation in those with chronic obstructive pulmonary disease.

Relaxation strategies:

These may include deep breathing, meditation, and biofeedback.

Education/Prevention

Healthy lifestyles, a good diet, and regular exercise decrease the likelihood of chronic disease. Stopping smoking, even later in life, can have a positive effect on respiratory status. Older adults are reminded to get influenza and pneumoccal vaccines.

CONTINUING EDUCATION

Self-Assessment Examination

How to Obtain Continuing Education Credit

Registered nurses may receive one contact hour by viewing the video, reviewing the accompanying booklet, and successfully answering the questions in the following post-test. You must answer 70% of the questions correctly to receive a passing grade. The post-test is designed to validate your understanding of the content.

Taking the Test

1. Read each test question and record your answer on the answer sheet provided. DO NOT DUPLICATE THIS ANSWER SHEET. A PHOTOCOPY WILL BE REJECTED BY THE SCANNER.

2. Follow the instructions on the answer sheet exactly. Use only a No. 2 pencil, and do not make any stray marks on the answer sheet. It is important that you PRINT your name, address, and Social Security number correctly; failure to do so will result in rejection of your answer sheet by the computer.

3. Forward the completed answer sheet to:

Mosby, Inc.
Division of Continuing Education & Training
Attn: Geriatric Symptom Assessment and Management: Cardiopulmonary
11830 Westline Industrial Drive
St. Louis, MO 63146-3318

Continuing Education Credit

Mosby/Division of Continuing Education and Training (DCET) is an approved provider of continuing education in nursing by the American Nurses Credentialing Center Commission on Accreditation. This approval is reciprocal in all states and for all specialty organizations who recognize the ANCC approval process.

Mosby/DCET is also an approved provider of nursing continuing education in: Iowa—No. 133 Board of Nursing Criteria 5.3(2)a(1,2,5); Provider approved by the California Board of Registered Nursing, Provider No. 03257.

Mosby/DCET contact hours are applicable for recertification/relicensure requirements for all professional associations and in all states requiring mandatory continuing education that recognize the ANCC approval process.

Receiving Your Results

Your post-test will be graded and the results forwarded by postcard within 90 days of receipt of your completed answer sheet.

PLEASE KEEP THE POSTCARD; IT IS YOUR CERTIFICATE OF CONTACT HOURS EARNED.

If you have any questions related to the test or your results, call 800-826-1877.

POST-TEST

1. Which statement is *false* about the composition of water in the older adult?
   a. It is reduced to 45 percent of total body weight.
   b. Two-thirds of fluid is intracellular.
   c. It is increased by 10 percent with normal aging.
   d. The extracellular proportion is greater with increased age.

2. Starling's concept of osmotic pressure shows that:
   a. fluid flows from the vessel in response to intravascular pressure.
   b. fluid flows from the vessel in response to the colloid pressure of the interstitial fluid.
   c. fluid enters the blood because of interstitial tissue tension.
   d. fluid enters the blood because of the oncotic pressure of protein.
   e. all of the above.

3. Edema caused by a dietary insufficiency of protein is a result of:
   a. excess sodium retention.
   b. increased interstitial volume.
   c. increased intravascular oncotic pressure.
   d. decrease in sodium levels.

4. The most effective way of measuring fluid accumulation is:
   a. use of an edema scale.
   b. serial weights of the older adult.
   c. anthropometric skin fold measurements.
   d. sodium level measurement.

5. The most common symptoms of myocardial infarction in those over age 85 are:
   a. chest pain and diaphoresis.
   b. edema and chest discomfort.
   c. shortness of breath and confusion.

6. Unstable chest pain must be evaluated immediately in the hospital. Examples of unstable pain include:
   a. recent onset.
   b. recent change in the frequency or severity.
   c. rest angina.
   d. all of the above.

7. Auscultation of the valvular areas of the heart is best done with the:
   a. diaphragm, because heart sounds are high frequency.
   b. the bell, because heart sounds are low frequency.
   c. both the diaphragm and the bell.

8. When gastroesophageal reflux disease is the etiology of chest discomfort, the best nonpharmacological strategy would include:
   a. fewer meals.
   b. over-the-counter antacid therapy.
   c. keeping the head elevated after meals.
   d. an after-dinner mint.

9. Proper technique for diaphragmatic breathing includes:
    a. tightening the abdomen during inspiration, relaxing with expiration.
    b. pursing the lips to increase airway resistance.
    c. relaxing the abdomen during inspiration, tightening with expiration.
    d. pursing the lips to decrease airway resistance.

CASE STUDY 1

Sadie Foster, 84, is a new participant in the adult day care center. She has Alzheimer's disease and attends the center three days a week. On her admission nursing assessment, you note she has some mild pitting edema in her lower extremeties that is equal bilaterally. Her skin is dry, turgor poor. Mrs. Foster is unable to give a history, and her daughter reports she has been eating poorly for several weeks and has lost 10 pounds in three months. The family is hopeful that the social atmosphere at the center will stimulate her appetite. She has no significant history except for arthritis, for which she is given Motrin 400 milligrams two times daily.

What may be contributing to Mrs. Foster's edema?

CASE STUDY 2

Alice Rodriguez, 71, presents in the emergency room after 2 hours of severe substernal chest pain. She reported several episodes of activity-induced angina over the last three months, relieved with rest or nitroglycerine. This time, the pain started without provocation and did not respond to several sublingual nitroglycerine tabs. Past medical history is significant for hypertension and type 2 diabetes mellitus. On admission to the chest pain center, EKG showd atrial fibrillation and 3 mm ST segment elevation in leads V1 and V4. She was diagnosed with an acute anterior wall MI, and her cardiac catherization revealed an occlusion of the LAD. After balloon catheter inflations, the blood flow was restored and the artery remained patent. At this point, her atrial fibrillation converted to normal sinus rhythm and the ST segment elevation had almost completely resolved.

What health teaching strategies are important?

CASE STUDY 3

Chuck Peters is your 75-year-old grandfather who calls you complaining of mild shortness of breath and fatigue. You are concerned and do a home visit to assess the situation since he was not very specific with details on the phone. You find your grandfather in mild distress due to dyspnea (respiratory rate is 22). He has crackles in his bases bilaterally, he has no neck vein distension, and he has a third heart sound. He has no edema, and his abdominal exam is negative. Past medical history is essentially negative, although he has smoked two packs of cigarettes per day for 40 years, and he continues to do so. He was recently diagnosed as having glaucoma. He is evaluated in the emergency room; the diagnosis is mild heart failure. The precipitant is the beta blocker in the eyedrop he was given for the glaucoma. He recovers fully after a short course of diuretic therapy.

What is the pathophysiological mechanism that contributed to his heart failure?

REFERENCES

Edema

Abrams WB, Beers MH, Berkow R: *The Merck manual of geriatrics*, ed 2, Whitehouse Station, NJ, 1995, Merck Research Laboratories.

Ciocon JO, Fernandez BB, Ciocon DG: Leg edema: clinical clues to the differential diagnosis, *Geriatrics* 48:34-45, 1993.

DeGowin RL: *DeGowin and DeGowin's bedside diagnostic examination*, ed 5, New York, 1987, Macmillan Publishing Company.

Galindo-Ciocon D: Nursing care of elders with leg edema, *Journal of Gerontological Nursing* 21(7):7-11, 1995.

Martin PY, Schrier RW: Renal sodium excretion and edematous disorders, *Endocrinology and Metabolism Clinics of North America* 24(3):459-479, 1995.

Merli G, Spandorfer J: The outpatient with unilateral leg swelling, *Medical Clinics of North America* 79(2):435-447, 1995.

Streeten D: Idiopathic edema: pathogenesis, clinical features, and treatment, *Endocrinology and Metabolism Clinics of North America* 24(3):531-547, 1995.

Chest Pain

Aisenberg J, Castell D: Approach to the patient with unexplained chest pain, *Mount Sinai Journal of Medicine* 61(6):476-483, 1994.

Bayer AJ, Chadha JS, Farag RR: Changing presentation of myocardial infarction with increasing old age, *Journal of the American Geriatrics Association* 34:263-266, 1986.

Bittner V, Clark DM: Chest pain of unknown origin: the differential diagnosis, *Hospital Medicine* July: 12-19, 1995.

Howell J, Hedges JR: Differential diagnosis of chest comfort and general approach to myocardial ischemia decision making, *American Journal of Emergency Medicine* 9(6):571-579, 1991.

Limacher M: Chapter 6: Clinical features of coronary heart disease in the elderly. In Lowenthal D, ed. *Geriatric cardiology*, Philadelphia, F. A. Davis Company.

Singh S, Richter JE, Bradley LA, Haile J: The symptom index: differential usefulness in suspected acid-related complaints of heartburn and chest pain, *Digestive Diseases and Sciences* 38(8):1402-1488, 1993.

Wasson J, Walsh BT, Tompkins R, Sox H, Pantell R: *The common symptom guide*, ed 3, New York, 1992, McGraw Hill.

Williams B: Chapter 25: Chest pain. In Martin A, Camm AJ, eds. *Geriatric cardiology: principles and practice*, Chichester, NY, 1994, John Wiley and Sons Ltd.

Dyspnea

Borg GAV: Psychophysical basis of perceived exertion, *Med Sci Sports Exerc* 14:380, 1982.

Gift AG, Pugh LC: Dyspnea and fatigue, *Nursing Clinics of North America* 28(2):373-383, 1993.

Mahler DA: Dyspnea: diagnosis and management, *Clin Chest Med* 8:224, 1987.

Raffin TA: Approach to the patient with dyspnea, *Hospital Medicine* October: 45-65, 1984.

Seamens CM, Wrean K: Breathlessness, *Postgraduate Medicine* 98(4):215-227, 1995.

Seidel HM, Ball JW, Dains JE, Benedict GW: *Mosby's guide to physical examination*, St Louis, 1991, Mosby, Inc.

Silvestri GA, Mahler DA: Evaluation of dyspnea in the elderly patient, *Clinics in Chest Medicine* 14(3):393-404, 1993.

TABLES

Table 2-1 Cardiopulmonary Changes with Aging
With permission from Stone JT, Wyman J: *Clinical gerontological nursing: guidelines for advanced practice*, ed 2, Philadelphia, In Press, WB Saunders.

FIGURES

Figure 2-4 Possible Causes of Chest Pain of Unkown Origin
Redrawn with permission from Bittner V, Clark DM: Chest pain of unknown origin: the differential diagnosis, *Hospital Medicine* July:12-19, 1995.

Figure 2-5 Valvular Areas
With permission from Seidel HM, Ball JW, Dains JE, Benedict GW: *Mosby's guide to physical examination*, St. Louis, 1991, Mosby, Inc.

Figure 2-6 Factors Influencing the Control of Ventilation
Redrawn with permission from Raffin TA: Approach to the patient with dyspnea, *Hospital Medicine* October: 46-65, 1984.

Figure 2-7 Dyspnea in Cardiac Failure
Redrawn with permission from Raffin TA: Approach to the patient with dyspnea, *Hospital Medicine* October: 46-65, 1984.

Figure 2-8 Dyspnea Scales
Redrawn with permission from Mahler DA: Dyspnea: diagnosis and management, *Clin Chest Med* 8:224, 1987.

Redrawn with permission from Borg GAV: Psychophysical basis of perceived exertion, *Med Sci Sports Exerc* 14:380, 1982.

Figure 2-9 Schema of Breath Sounds in the Well and Ill Patient
With permission from Seidel HM, Ball JW, Dains JE, Benedict GW: *Mosby's guide to physical examination*, St. Louis, 1991, Mosby, Inc.

Figure 2-10 Clubbing
With permission from Seidel HM, Ball JW, Dains JE, Benedict GW: *Mosby's guide to physical examination*, St. Louis, 1991, Mosby, Inc.